THE IBS SLOW COOKER COOKBOOK

50 Low FODMAP Slow Cooker Recipes To Relieve Symptoms of IBS

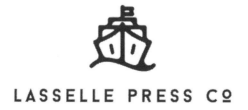

LASSELLE PRESS CO

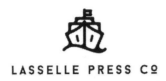

LASSELLE PRESS Co

ISBN-13: 978-1911364481
ISBN-10: 1911364480

CONTENTS

INTRODUCTION

Welcome to The IBS Slow Cooker Cookbook!

We understand that experiencing the symptoms of IBS can be extremely uncomfortable and even very painful. We also know that for some it may be embarrassing to share your experiences of IBS with those around you, due to the very nature of the syndrome. This book has been written in order to help you understand more about the syndrome as well as provide you with 50 low Fodmap recipes that can be made with ease, and left to cook while you sleep or go about your daily activities! Our intention is to take a little of the stress and anxiety away from the cooking, so that you can focus on eating well and feeling better.

It may be you or someone you know who suffers from IBS, or it's possible that you suspect you may be experiencing the symptoms and would like to know more about it. Either way, it is extremely important that you consult your doctor if you notice any of the symptoms outlined later in this book. We hope that reading this can give you the confidence to go and discuss your symptoms and concerns with a professional, if you haven't done so already.

Along with information about IBS and the possible symptoms and causes, this book provides detailed lists of low Fodmap foods to be enjoyed, as well as those to avoid. The shopping, eating out and travel guidance chapter aims to help you get on with things in the way you deserve to.

We understand that it is unlikely that everyone in the family will suffer from IBS and therefore we offer hints and tips as you go along for bulk cooking, storage and freezing portions. That being said, we only use fresh and healthy ingredients in these recipes and each dish provides a balance of healthy fats, carbohydrates, proteins and vitamins, so all the family can enjoy the recipes provided! The nutritional values of each recipe are calculated, in order to help you plan your meals and keep track of what you're eating. Hopefully this will take the strain out of meal planning and preparation, and allow you and the family to enjoy dinner time again!

We wish you all the best in the kitchen and in health!
The Lasselle Press Team

C1: IBS OVERVIEW

IBS affects the large intestine and can cause changes and discomfort during bowel movements. These range in severity from person to person and can be inconvenient, uncomfortable and sometimes even debilitating. Unfortunately the syndrome is incurable, but it can be managed with long term treatment, diet and lifestyle choices.

The exact cause of IBS is unknown, however it may be caused by a problem in the interaction between the gut, the brain and the nervous system. Some factors, such as stress, can worsen symptoms of IBS whilst they do not cause it. Surprisingly very few people seek medical help despite suffering from the symptoms of IBS; in the US, most patients finally seek help around six years after the symptoms of IBS start. It is essential that you do seek a professional diagnosis of IBS if you are concerned that you may be experiencing the symptoms of the syndrome, or if you have a family history of IBS.

According to www.aboutibs.org, 'IBS affects between 25 and 45 million people in the United States.' Of these, two thirds are female. IBS can affect people of all age ranges but is most prevalent in those under 50 years old and can also affect children. Unfortunately it is a syndrome that many are embarrassed to get help for or talk about with their peers due to the nature of the syndrome's symptoms. Thus many end up worsening their symptoms through not getting suitable help and guidance. Treatments are available to help manage IBS and as previously mentioned, changes in your diet and lifestyle can help lessen symptoms which vary from person to person.

So don't lose hope if you've recently been diagnosed, or think you might be suffering from IBS. Seek medical opinion, talk to a trusted family member or friend, and know that there are things that can be changed in order to relieve the pain and discomfort you may be currently feeling.

Symptoms of IBS

There are a variety of symptoms associated with IBS and these can often coincide. These include:

• Diarrhoea
• Constipation
• Abdominal pain and cramping
• Gas
• Feeling bloated
• Mucus in the stool

You should seek out medical help if you develop symptoms of rectal bleeding, abdominal pain that becomes severely worse at night, or unexplained weight loss. These are symptoms that could worsen the overall effects of IBS, or could point to more serious underlying issues with your health.

There are two categories of IBS:

IBS-D - resulting in diarrhoea symptoms.

IBS-C - resulting in constipation symptoms.

Although there are two categories, it is important to remember that your symptoms can alternate and shift between the two.

IBS Triggers

Although as previously mentioned, the exact cause of IBS is unknown, we know how it occurs in comparison to a healthy intestinal tract system in a person without IBS: layers of muscle line the walls of our intestines that either contract or relax in order to move the food we consume from our stomach all the way down to our rectum, through the intestinal tract. With IBS, these contractions may either be stronger, lasting longer than usual, thus causing gas, bloating, and diarrhoea, or they may be weaker and slower than usual, thus causing constipation.
There are many different triggers for the symptoms of IBS to occur; these range from person to person, and can also change over time for a particular individual. It is important to keep all possible triggers in mind because of IBS being a terribly unpredictable syndrome. Some of the most common triggers are:

- Specific foods - this can vary between individuals.
  Food allergies or intolerances e.g. chocolate, spices, fat, beans, fruits, cauliflower, cabbage, broccoli, milk, soda, carbonated drinks, alcohol etc.
- Stress - triggers an over-active nervous system which can intensify the signals sent to the gastrointestinal area of the body and cause stronger contractions.
- Hormones - particularly worsening during a woman's menstrual cycle.
- Other illnesses e.g. anxiety or depression.
  Excess intestinal bacteria - can interfere with the digestion process and contribute to IBS symptoms.

Other Conditions Linked To IBS

What makes diagnosing and treating IBS a little complicated is that there are other conditions and diseases which are linked to the syndrome. These can produce similar symptoms and in some cases worsen IBS symptoms. Please discuss these conditions and symptoms with your doctor in order to receive suitable and specific treatment.

SIBO - a condition linked to and associated with IBS. SIBO stands for Small Intestine Bacteria Overgrowth. This overgrowth can interfere with the digestion process and absorption of food as well as damage the membrane lining. It is healthy to have a certain amount of bacteria in our gut. In this case however, there will be an excessive amount of bacteria; this can cause chronic fatigue, body pains, and stress on the liver. Through the damage caused to the membrane lining, larger food particles are able to pass through without being properly digested; this can cause food allergies and sensitivities. If you are diagnosed and treated for SIBO, your IBS symptoms may also be alleviated.

Celiac Disease - another condition linked to IBS. Celiac Disease causes a sensitivity to gluten. Gluten is a protein that is contained in barley, rye, and wheat products. Celiac disease can cause symptoms such as anemia, fatigue, diarrhoea, bloating and weight loss, which can sometimes lead to serious complications. Celiac disease can worsen IBS symptoms.

In the next chapter we will discuss dietary and lifestyle changes you can make in order to help relieve the symptoms of IBS.

C2: DIET AND LIFESTYLE GUIDANCE

Along with the treatment prescribed by your doctor and their guidance, making changes to your diet and lifestyle can have an extremely positive effect on your symptoms and your lifestyle. There are a number of different diets that have been recommended for IBS sufferers and each person will react differently to certain foods, so it is important to bear this in mind. Be mindful of which foods trigger your symptoms as well as those that do not; you can do this by keeping a journal of the foods and drinks you eat as well as your symptoms experienced daily. This method will allow you to notice if there are any patterns with certain foods or ingredients that may be triggering symptoms.

This cookbook uses low FODMAP foods as the diet that is most commonly now recommended for those with IBS. Again, this may vary from patient to patient and it is imperative to seek dietary guidance from a professional before changing your diet. Information about the low FODMAP diet will be given in the next section so that you can find out more about it.

The Low FODMAP Diet

FODMAPs stand for Fermentable, Oligio-, Di-, Mono-saccharides And Polyols. FODMAPs are carbohydrates with short chains that naturally occur in food and are not properly absorbed through the small intestine. Choosing foods and portion sizes that are low in FODMAPs can greatly reduce the triggering of symptoms.

- Use the lists on the following pages to select foods and portion sizes that are classed as Low FODMAP.
- Avoid those that are classed as high FODMAP.

Please note, whilst some foods may be classed as low FODMAP, this can depend on the portion size. Take note of the portion sizes for each type of food and ingredient so that you don't go over the recommended serving sizes.

Fruits:
LOW FODMAP - Enjoy (stick to 1 fruit/1 cup per serving whichever is the smaller quantity):
Banana (1/2 large banana serving/approx. 30g),
Blueberries – buy organic,
Boysenberry – buy organic,
Cantaloupe,
Star fruit,
Cranberry – buy organic,
Durian, Grapes – buy organic,
Grapefruit,
Honeydew melon,
Kiwi,
Lemon,
Lime,
Mandarin,
Orange,
Passion fruit,
Paw Paw,
Pineapple,
Raspberry – buy organic,
Rhubarb,
Strawberry – buy organic,
Tangelo.

HIGH FODMAP - Avoid - (any fruits of more than 1 cup per serving) plus:
Apple,
Mango,
Nashi Fruit,
Pear,
Persimmon,
Watermelon,
Persimmon,
Rambutan,
Apricot,
Avocado,
Blackberries,
Cherries,

Longon,
Lychee,
Nectarine,
Peach,
Plum,
Prune.

VEGETABLES: Enjoy (stick to 1 vegetable/1 cup per serving whichever is the smaller quantity):
Alfalfa,
Bamboo Shoots,
Bean Shoots,
Beans (green),
Bok Choy,
Capsicum,
Carrot (1 medium carrot),
Celery,
Chives (green section only),
Choy Sum,
Cucumber,
Endive,
Fennel heart (1 small heart or smaller 49g),
Ginger,
Lettuce (may be okay for some),
Marrow,
Olives,
Parsnip,
Parsley,
Potato (2 small potatoes),
Pumpkin (1/2 cup),
Silver beet,
Scallions (green section only),
Spinach (1 cup),
Swede,
Sweet potato (3 tbsp),
Taro,
Beef tomatoes,
Turnip,

Yam,
Eggplant,
Zucchini (this may be okay for some; check individual tolerance).

Avoid (any vegetables of more than 1 cup per serving) plus:
Artichokes (Globe and Jerusalem),
Asparagus,
Beets,
Broccoli,
Brussel Sprouts,
Cabbage,
Chicory,
Dandelion leaves,
Garlic,
Legumes, Okra, Onion (brown, white, and Spanish), Peas, Radicchio Lettuce, Shallots, Leeks, Scallions and Chives (white sections),
Squash ,
Cauliflower,
Mushrooms,
Snow peas and Sugar Snap Peas,
Corn,
Cherry Tomatoes (due to mould).
Please note: there is undeclared onion hidden in many processed foods including, chicken salt, vegetable salt, vegetable powder, dehydrated vegetables, stocks, gravies, soups, marinades, and sauces. Make sure you check ingredients labels for packaged items and avoid onion.

Flavorings and Herbs and Spices
Enjoy:
Pecans, Walnuts (max. 15 per serving),
Golden Syrup, Treacle, Molasses, Maple Syrup,
White, Brown, Raw and Castor Sugar,
Tea and Herbal Teas,
Seeds (in moderation),
Oat bran (max. 1/4 cup serving), Rolled Oats (max. 1/4 cup serving), Gluten Free Oats,
Barley Bran, Psyllium, Rice Bran,
Stevia, Baking Cocoa Powder, Carob Powder,
Olive Oil, Canola Oil, Garlic-infused Oil, Coconut Oil,

Unsweetened Desiccated Coconut (max. 1/4 cup serving),
Fresh and dried Ginger, Cilantro, Basil, Lemongrass, Mint, Parsley, Marjoram, Thyme, Rosemary and other herbs.

Avoid:
Honey, Corn syrups, Fruisana,
Chicory and Dandelion Tea,
Artificial Sweeteners,
Sugar free or Low Carb Sweets, Mints or Gums,
Dairy Desserts,
Baked Beans, Lentils, Chickpeas,
Solid Chocolate, Solid Carob, Olives,
Nuts and Nut Butters,
Caffeine, Decaf Coffee.

Dairy and Other
Enjoy:
Egg Whites,
Rice milk, Almond Milk, Raw Goats milk, Hemp milk,
Goats Cheese,
Cottage Cheese.

Avoid:
Other Cheeses,
Egg Yolks,
Dairy (Milk, Cream, Yogurt, Butter, Sour Cream),
Soy Milk, Coconut Milk,
Vegetable Oils.

Wheat Products and Alternatives:
Enjoy:
Rice, Amaranth, Tapioca, Quinoa, Millet, Sorghum, Buckwheat, Arrowroot, Sago,
Gluten Free (GF) Bread, Gluten Free Pasta,
Rice Noodles, Wheat Free Buckwheat Noodles,
Porridge, Wheat Free Muesli, Rice Bubbles, Gluten Free Cereals, Rice Cakes and Crackers, GF crackers, Ryvitas, and Rye Cruskits,
GF cakes, Flourless Cakes, GF biscuits, GF Pastry Mixes and Bread Crumbs,
Polenta, Buckwheat, Millet and Rice Flours.

Avoid:
Bread (white, wholemeal, multigrain, sourdough).
Pasta and Noodles (regular, two minute, spelt, egg noodles, hokkien and udon),
Breakfast Cereals (containing wheat, excess dried fruit and/or fruit juice),
Savory Biscuits (wheat based),
Cakes and Baked Goods (wheat based), Biscuits (wheat based),
Pastry and Breadcrumbs (wheat flour made),
Others (semolina, couscous, bulgur).

Protein Sources:
Enjoy:
Oily Fish,
Lean Meats e.g. Skinless Chicken or Turkey Breasts.

Avoid:
Red meat,
Dark Meat from Poultry e.g. turkey/chicken thighs,
Soy Products e.g. tofu/tempeh.

Lifestyle Guidance

Along with a diet that prevents or lessens the trigger of your IBS symptoms, other lifestyle changes can help you to feel healthier and less stressed, thus alleviating symptoms further.

1.   Ensure you exercise regularly - 20-30 minutes per day or 2-3 times per week will boost serotonin levels, helping you to feel happier and less stressed. Additionally you will feel great physically and prevent other serious illnesses such as obesity and heart disease.

2.   Eat your meals slowly and mindfully. In other words, not at your computer on a 'working lunch', rushing to pick up the kids, or on the way to work. This will help to prevent the symptoms such as cramps and bloating.

3.   Avoid chewing gum, especially when you're not eating soon after. The saliva that builds in your mouth sends a signal to your stomach that you are about to eat, if this is not the case it confuses the digestive system and can trigger symptoms.

4.   Drink plenty of water! This greatly improves general health as well as assisting the digestive system in flushing out slow to move particles and preventing constipation.

5.   Evaluate your work/life balance. Is the commute causing you unnecessary stress? Is there someone who can possibly help with the childcare or chores in any way? Can you cut down on unnecessary expenses so that you have more money to pay for childcare? Whatever helps prevent or cut down stress can have a dramatic positive effect on your symptoms.

6.   Try to get plenty of sleep by winding down at least one hour before you would like to be asleep and turning off all computers and electronic devices. Use an alarm clock rather than your phone and turn off anything electric at the wall; the blue lighting and signals can interfere with your brain waves and keep you alert when you want to be fast asleep!

7.   IBS can be a source of embarrassment to many sufferers and many end up

concealing their symptoms or avoiding situations because of them. IBS can really affect the way you get on with everyday life. Reach out to a local support group or to online forums if you don't want to discuss it with family and friends. Talk to your doctors for advice. If you can, tell someone at work who you feel you can trust so that you don't find yourself having to make up excuses for sick days or even mid shift. You will be surprised at how understanding your colleagues and employers can be!

8.   Consider therapies - counselling can be extremely helpful; as with any other physical or mental illness, IBS can cause mental and physical symptoms. Consider cognitive behavioural therapy, hypnotherapy, biofeedback and others. Your local support group, doctors or the internet may be able to help you work out what type of therapy would benefit you the most.

9.   Take a look at your medications - some medications prescribed to you may actually be worsening the symptoms of IBS including: antibiotics, some antidepressants, and medicine containing sorbitol such as cough syrups, prozac, sarafem and zoloft can cause diarrhoea. Speak to your doctor about any current medication you're on and whether they these can be adjusted to your needs. Always consult your doctor before discontinuing any medications.

C3: EATING OUT AND TRAVEL GUIDE
Advice for Dining Out

It can be very hard for you to dine out with friends and family if you suffer from IBS; you never know when your symptoms might be triggered and what foods may or may not be available. But you don't have to miss out on your favorite restaurant or cuisines! Here are a few tips that may make dining out easier for you:

- Research the restaurant's menu beforehand and decide what you will choose to avoid anxiety and spontaneous decisions on the night.
- Use the food lists in the previous chapter to help you choose and don't feel bad about asking the restaurant to cater to your needs.
- Ask your server for your foods to be cooked without extra salts, butters or sauces.
- Avoid fried foods and opt for grilled or poached instead.
- Avoid drinking alcohol and opt for water or lemonade instead.
- Eat slowly and pace yourself between courses.
- Take any medication you have been prescribed at the usual time.

Advice for traveling

1. Whatever your travel plans, you will have to eat. If you plan ahead, you should be able to make a meal plan that suits your need.
2. If you have a dietitian, tell them where you are going and what you expect to eat at your destination.
3. Remember to pack enough of any prescription medicines you must take.
4. If going on a road trip or camping, avoid processed meats and foods.
5. Take snacks suitable for the low FODMAP diet to avoid picking up treats from the service stations!
6. Do not consume dairy products.
7. If you are going on a cruise, all those buffet foods are tempting to eat 24 hours a day. To help with this predicament try to select fruits, salads, and vegetables from the low FODMAP lists.
8. Let the cruise line or hotel know of your dietary needs, most are willing to prepare special foods for you.
9. If you are going to be traveling abroad and don't speak the language, take a phrasebook that has a section for ordering food.
10. Check if you can check in early and check out late to avoid waiting around for flight times.

Cooking Tips

1. *Grill, poach, roast or sauté meats instead of frying.*
2. *Steam or boil vegetables instead of frying.*
3. *Use healthy oils such as extra virgin olive oil or coconut oil to shallow fry.*
4. *Avoid added sugars and opt for Stevia instead of sugar.*
5. *Herbs are more likely to calm the digestive system and your gut while spices are more likely to irritate it. Oregano, basil, parsley, sage, mint, thyme, cilantro, ginger, and cloves are great herbs to incorporate into your meals. You want to avoid spices like cayenne pepper, chili powder or any hot sauces.*

Useful Kitchen Equipment

- A selection of non-stick skillets,
- A large pot for soups and stews,
- A Slow Cooker,
- A set of Tupperware for storage and bulk cooking,
- Food Processor/blender/mortar and pestle
- Large Bowls for salads or mixing.

One Last Thing

Always remember to use new recipes and ingredients after speaking to your doctor or dietitian; your needs will be unique to you depending on your symptoms and the certain foods that trigger them.

We hope that with your doctor's advice, along with our guidance and recipes, that you can continue to enjoy cooking, eating and sharing meal times with your loved ones.

Thank you for purchasing this book and we wish you all the best on your path to health and contentment.

Happy cooking!

BREAKFAST

One-Pot Breakfast

SERVES 4 / PREP TIME: 10 MINUTES / COOK TIME: 4 HOURS LOW

A delicious burst of energy to kick-start the day.

---

1 tbsp olive oil
2 white potatoes, peeled and sliced
1/2 red bell pepper diced
12 egg whites
1 cup almond milk
A pinch of salt and pepper

1 green onion stem, finely sliced (green section only)
8 oz crumbled goats cheese

---

1. Lightly rub the bottom of the slow cooker pan with oil.
2. Add half the potato slices followed by half the peppers.
3. Beat the egg whites and the milk together.
4. Season the liquid with a little salt and pepper to taste.
5. Add in the green onion and stir.
6. Pour the egg mixture into the pot over the potatoes.
7. Cook everything on Low for 4 hours.
8. In the last ten minutes, crumble on the goats cheese.
9. Enjoy a hearty breakfast.

Per serving: Calories: 366 Protein: 22g Carbs: 23g Fiber: 2g Sugar: 6g Fat: 20g (Unsaturated: 8g Saturated: 12g)

Sweet and Soft Raspberry Rice Pudding

SERVES 4 / PREP TIME: 10 MINUTES / COOK TIME: 1 HOUR HIGH

Sweet, juicy and warming. Perfect.

1/2 cup short grain rice
1 ½ tbsp chia seeds
2 cups water
3 cups almond milk
1/2 tsp ground cinnamon
Maple syrup to taste (optional)
2 cups organic raspberries

---

1. Combine the rice, chia seeds, water, almond milk, and cinnamon in the slow cooker. Mix well.
2. Cook on High for 1 hour.
3. Stir halfway through if you can.
4. Once the rice is thick and creamy, remove from the pot.
5. Place to one side and allow to cool for a few minutes.
6. Taste and stir in some maple syrup if desired.
7. Stir in the raspberries 15 minutes before serving.

Hint: If you have time, cook on Low for 4-5 hours instead for a really smooth, rich flavor.

Per serving: Calories: 216 Protein: 4g Carbs: 41g Fiber: 7g Sugar: 14g Fat: 4g (Unsaturated: 4g Saturated: 0g)

Sweetened Slow Oats

SERVES 3 / PREP TIME: 5 MINUTES / COOK TIME: 5 HOURS LOW

Just a great breakfast classic.

---

1 tsp coconut oil
1 cup steel-cut oats
2 cups almond milk
½ cup water
1/2 cup raisins
2 tbsp maple syrup
1 tbsp cinnamon

---

1. Rub the inside of your slow cooker with coconut oil.
2. Add all ingredients to the slow cooker – nice and simple.
3. Cook on Low for 5 hours.
4. Serve warm with a little dusting of extra cinnamon on top.

Hint: Soak your raisins for a few hours in warm water beforehand to plump them up. 8 tablespoons of raisins per serving are classed as low FODMAP.

Per serving: Calories: 273 Protein: 5g Carbs: 55g Fiber 6g: Sugar: 29g Fat: 5g (Unsaturated: 3g Saturated: 2g)

Fruity Quinoa Porridge

SERVES 4 / PREP TIME: 5 MINUTES / COOK TIME: 2 HOURS HIGH

Similar to oat porridge but with a slightly chunkier texture and higher in protein.

---

1 cup dry quinoa
3 cups almond milk
2 tsp cinnamon
1/4 tsp nutmeg
1 tsp vanilla extract
1 tsp brown sugar
1/4 tsp salt
2 medium bananas, sliced
1 cup organic blueberries

---

1. Throw all the ingredients (apart from the fresh fruit) into a slow cooker.
2. Cook on High for 2 hours or until all the liquid is absorbed.
3. Serve with the fresh fruit on top.

Hint: Alternatively, you can cook this on Low overnight for 7-8 hours to have it ready in the morning.

Per serving: Calories: 306 Protein: 7g Carbs: 60g Fiber: 7g Sugar: 24g Fat: 5g (Unsaturated: 5g Saturated: 30)

Greek Red Pepper and Goats Cheese Frittata

SERVES 6 / PREP TIME: 10 MINUTES / COOK TIME: 3 HOURS LOW

Bold Greek-inspired flavors; pair with a green salad!

1 tbsp olive oil
12 oz roasted red peppers, drained and cut into small pieces
½ cup pitted black olives, sliced
8 egg whites, beaten
1 tsp dried basil

4 oz crumbled goats cheese
1/4 cup sliced green onions (green tips only)
Fresh ground black pepper to taste

1. Rub the inside of the slow cooker with olive oil.
2. Add the red peppers and olives to the pot.
3. Whisk the egg whites with the basil and pour over the vegetables.
4. Using a fork, gently stir the mixture.
5. Sprinkle the crumbled cheese over the top.
6. Cook on Low for 3 hours or until the eggs are firm.
7. Cut into pieces while the frittata is still in the slow cooker.
8. Serve hot, sprinkled with chopped green onions.
9. Sprinkle with black pepper if desired.

Hint: As a rule of thumb, eggs are best when cooked as slowly as possible.

Per serving: Calories: 134 Protein: 8g Carbs: 6g Fiber: 1g Sugar: 3g Fat: 9g (Unsaturated: 5g Saturated: 4g)

Home Baked Pecan Loaf

SERVES 8 / PREP TIME: 10 MINUTES / COOK TIME: 1 HOUR

Not a slow cooker recipe but a staple you will probably want to have in your recipe bank!

Coconut oil as needed
1 1/2 cups rice flour
1/2 cup buckwheat flour
3 tsp baking powder
1/2 tsp salt

2 tbsp coconut sugar
2 egg whites
1 cup unsweetened almond milk
1/2 cup coconut oil
2 tbsp crushed pecan nuts

---

1. Preheat the oven to 350 degrees.
2. Grease a loaf pan generously with coconut oil.
3. Sift together the rice flour, the buckwheat flour, the baking powder, and the salt into a large bowl.
4. Stir in the sugar.
5. Meanwhile, using an electric mixer, lightly beat the egg whites until they are just frothy.
6. Stir in the milk and the coconut oil.
7. Now pour the flour mixture into the bowl with the egg white mixture.
8. Beat on a medium speed for 2 to 3 minutes, or until smooth.
9. Pour this mixture into the greased loaf pan.
10. Smooth the top with a spatula.
11. Next, sprinkle the crushed pecans over the top of the mixture, pressing them down slightly.
12. Bake for 55 minutes to 1 hour, testing to see if a toothpick or knife comes out clean.
13. Set the pan to cool on a wire rack for at least 10 minutes.
14. Turn the bread out onto the wire rack to finish cooling.

Hint: You can substitute other gluten free flours in place of the rice and buckwheat flours depending on what you have in your cupboards!

Per serving: Calories: 268   Protein: 6g Carbs: 37g Sugar: 3g Fat: 18g

POULTRY

Rich Coq au Vin Stew

SERVES 6 / PREP TIME: 10 MINUTES / COOK TIME: 6 HOURS LOW

A classic French-inspired stew with warming flavors.

Olive oil cooking spray
16 oz chicken breasts, skinless and boneless
1 cup red wine
2 cups water
1 cup diced carrot
½ cup sliced green onion, (green tips only)
2 tbsp dried oregano
2 whole bay leaves
½ tsp dried thyme
½ cup low FODMAP chicken stock
2 tbsp tomato paste

1. Spray a large skillet with cooking oil, over medium heat.
2. Add the chicken and brown it evenly, turning occasionally.
3. Remove the chicken and add to the bottom of your slow cooker.
4. Use 1/2 of the red wine to de-glaze the skillet.
5. (Hint: Make sure to scrape up all the brown bits – that's the good stuff.)
6. Pour the wine from the skillet into the slow cooker.
7. Add the remaining wine, water, vegetables, herbs, stock and paste.
8. Stir to evenly distribute the ingredients in the slow cooker.
9. Cover and cook on Low 6 hours until the chicken and vegetables are tender.
10. Remove bay leaves before serving.

Per serving: Calories: 178 Protein: 24g Carbs: 6g Fiber: 2g Sugar: 2g Fat: 3g (Unsaturated: 2g Saturated: 1g)

Wild Rice and Chicken Stock

SERVES 4 / PREP TIME: 5 MINUTES / COOK TIME: 4 HOURS + 30 MINUTES HIGH

A slow cooking winter warming stock with an added flair.

---

4 carrots, peeled and chopped
1 large zucchini, chopped
16oz boneless, skinless chicken breasts, halved
1 tbsp unsalted butter
1/2 tsp dried oregano
1 bay leaf
4 cups low FODMAP chicken stock
1 cup water

3/4 cup wild rice
1 tsp garlic-infused olive oil
1 green onion, (green tips only), sliced
3 tbsp lemon juice
A pinch of salt and black pepper to taste
1 tbsp chopped fresh Italian parsley for serving

---

1. Add the first 8 ingredients to a large slow cooker.
2. Cook until the chicken is cooked through and the rice is tender (4 hours on High).
3. Transfer the chicken breasts to a cutting board and allow to cool slightly.
4. Meanwhile, heat the butter in a skillet on medium heat.
5. Add the onion and sauté until tender for 6 to 8 minutes.
6. Shred the chicken with a knife and fork and add it back to the slow cooker with the onion.
7. Cover and cook until the chicken is heated through (30 minutes on High).
8. Add water or stock to thin to your desired consistency.
9. Turn off the slow cooker and stir in the lemon juice.
10. Season to taste with salt and black pepper.
11. Ladle into bowls and top with fresh parsley.

Per serving: Calories: 254 Protein:28g Carbs: 17g Fiber: 2g Sugar: 4g Fat: 8g (Unsaturated: 6g Saturated: 2g)

Tender Turkey Wraps

SERVES 8 / PREP TIME: 10 MINUTES / COOK TIME: 7 HOURS LOW

Nice and healthy and packed with flavor.

---

1 lb turkey breasts, skinless and boneless
14.5 oz can low sodium diced tomatoes
1 cup water
1 tbsp dried parsley
3/4 tbsp sea salt
1/4 tbsp black pepper
8 6" rice/corn tortillas
2 cups pineapple chunks (or 1 can Dole sliced pineapple)

1 cup raw spinach, washed
1/4 cup fresh cilantro, chopped

Lime dressing:

1/4 cup lime juice
1/4 cup olive oil
1/2 tsp sugar
1/4 tsp salt

---

1. Spray the bottom of your slow cooker with cooking spray.
2. Place the turkey breasts in the cooker.
3. Add in the tomatoes, water, parsley, salt and pepper. Stir to combine.
4. Cover and cook on Low for 7 hours.
5. Prepare the lime dressing by mixing all the ingredients, cover and chill in the refrigerator.
6. After 7 hours, carefully remove the turkey with meat claws and shred (alternatively use two forks) and place to one side.
7. With a spoon, top each tortilla with 1/8 cup the turkey meat.
8. Divide the pineapple among the tortillas.
9. Toss the spinach and the cilantro with the lime dressing.
10. Top the tortillas with the salad and wrap into neat parcels.

Hint: There will be a nice thick sauce in the bottom of the slow cooker - use in the wraps if desired.

Per serving: Calories: 199 Protein: 14g Carbs: 19g Fiber: 3g Sugar: 6g Fat: 8g (Unsaturated: 7g Saturated: 1g)

Slow Cooker Turkey Masala Curry

SERVES 4 / PREP TIME: 10 MINUTES / COOK TIME: 1 HOUR 45 MINUTES LOW

Soft, juicy and delicately spiced.

---

1 lb skinless and boneless turkey breasts, cut into 2" slices
1 (14.5 oz) can diced tomatoes
1 tsp curry powder
1 tsp garam masala
1 tsp salt
1/2 tsp Asafoetida Powder
1/4 tsp dried cilantro

1/2 cup dairy-free sour cream/yogurt (optional)

---

1. Add all the ingredients (except the sour cream) into a food processor.
2. Grind until fully blended.
3. Add your spice mixture to the slow cooker.
4. Add your turkey slices. Cover.
5. Cook on Low for 1 hour 45 minutes until turkey is thoroughly cooked through.
6. Add the sour cream/yoghurt and swirl through.
7. Serve with rice if desired.

Per serving: Calories: 185 Protein: 25g Carbs: 7g Fiber: 1g Sugar: 0g Fat: 6g (Unsaturated: 0g Saturated: 5g)

Turkey-Stuffed Red Peppers

SERVES 6 / PREP TIME: 15 MINUTES / COOK TIME: 7-8 HOURS LOW

Tasty, herby and rich with melting cheese.

1 lb lean ground turkey
1 cup uncooked white rice
8 oz goats cheese, crumbled
1 tbsp diced chives
1 tsp salt
1/2 tsp ground black pepper
1 tsp dried rosemary
6 large red bell peppers, tops cut off
and de-seeded

Sauce:

32 oz fresh beef tomatoes, diced and
juices reserved
2 tsp minced fresh parsley
1 tsp dried oregano
1 tsp brown sugar
A pinch of baking soda
1 ½ cups low FODMAP vegetable stock

1. Mix together the first 7 ingredients for the stuffing.
2. Stuff evenly into the peppers, about 3/4 of the way full.
3. Spray the inside of your slow cooker with cooking oil.
4. Place the stuffed peppers inside.
5. Combine the first 5 ingredients of the sauce.
6. Pour this sauce over the peppers, then pour the stock around the sides into the base of the slow cooker pan.
7. Cover and cook on Low for 7 to 8 hours.

Per serving: Calories: 382 Protein: 25g Carbs: 26g Fiber: 2g Sugar: 7g Fat: 20g (Unsaturated: 9g Saturated: 10g)

Hearty Turkey and Vegetable Casserole

SERVES 4 / PREP TIME: 10 MINUTES / COOK TIME: 8 HOURS LOW

Wonderfully warming with chunky vegetables.

1½ cups leek (green tips only)
3 cups parsnip, peeled and cubed
2 large carrots
10 oz potatoes, peeled and cubed
12 oz lean turkey breasts, skinless and boneless
1 tbsp olive oil
1 tsp dried oregano

1/2 tsp dried thyme
4 cups low FODMAP chicken stock
1 cup boiling water
1 tbsp ground black pepper
6oz green beans
3 tbsp fresh parsley

1. Spray the bottom of your slow cooker dish with cooking oil.
2. Turn the cooker onto the Low setting.
3. Roughly chop the leeks, parsnips, carrots and potatoes into cubes.
4. Add the turkey to the slow cooker.
5. Add the vegetables.
6. Add the olive oil, dried oregano and thyme.
7. Pour the stock into the slow cooker.
8. Add the boiling water along with the black pepper.
9. Leave the slow cooker to cook on Low for 8 hours.
10. Check the stew after this time – if a little bit dry, add some boiling water until the ingredients are just covered.
11. Trim the green beans.
12. Blanch in a small saucepan for 2 to 3 minutes until tender.
13. Stir them through the stew.
14. Divide the stew into bowls and garnish with fresh parsley. Enjoy!

Per serving: Calories: 387 Protein: 27g Carbs: 52g Fiber: 10g Sugar: 10g Fat: 9g (Unsaturated: 7g Saturated: 2g)

Chicken Meatballs with Fluffy Rice

SERVES 8 / PREP TIME: 10 MINUTES / COOK TIME: 3 HOURS LOW/1.5 HOURS HIGH

Tender, juicy meatballs in a tangy tomato sauce.

---

1 celery stick, sliced
2 small carrots, peeled and sliced
4 5oz skinless chicken breasts, sliced
2 tbsp chives (green tips only)
1 tbsp olive oil, for greasing
1 cup tomato paste
1 cup low FODMAP chicken stock

1 cup beef tomatoes, sliced
2 cups cooked white rice

---

1. Blend the celery, carrots, chicken and chives in a food processor.
2. Shape into small meatballs with the palms of your hands.
3. To cook, grease the slow cooker with olive oil.
4. Add the meatballs, tomato paste and chicken stock to combine.
5. Cook on High for 3 hours on Low or 1 1/2 hours on High.
6. Add the fresh tomatoes 15 minutes before serving.
7. Served with freshly cooked rice.

Tip: This is a high protein dish so please keep track of your daily protein intake compared to the average recommendations – this will make up 50% of this amount! Great if you're working out, or not getting much protein from your other meals.

Per serving: Calories: 220 Protein: 24.5g Carbs: 20g Fiber: 2.5g Sugar:5.5g Fat: 5g (Unsaturated: 4g Saturated: 1g)

Italian-Seasoned Chicken Bake

SERVES 8 / PREP TIME: 15 MINUTES / COOK TIME: 5 HOURS LOW

Very easy and delicious, sure to be a weekly favorite.

---

1 tbsp olive oil
4 5oz skinless chicken breasts
1 stick of celery, finely chopped
1 carrot, peeled and finely diced
14 oz fresh beef tomatoes, quartered
1 cup low FODMAP chicken stock
1 tbsp tomato paste

1 tbsp garlic-infused oil
1 tsp brown sugar
1 tbsp fresh basil, torn
A pinch of salt and pepper
1lb 5oz potatoes, peeled and cubed
1 tbsp chopped fresh chives (green tips only) to garnish

---

1. Heat a large saucepan over medium heat.
2. Add the oil and, once hot, add the chicken breasts.
3. Brown the chicken for about 3-4 minutes, or until golden-brown.
4. Remove from the pan and add to the slow cooker.
5. Add the celery and carrot and stir.
6. Pour over the tomatoes, stock, paste, garlic oil, sugar and basil.
7. Mix well to make sure everything is evenly distributed.
8. Season with a little salt and pepper if desired.
9. Cover with a lid and cook on Low for 5 hours.
10. Add the potatoes with one hour to go.
11. Serve with a scatter of chives.

Hint: As this meal serves 8, portion up the leftovers and freeze in an airtight container for 2-3 weeks.

Per serving: Calories: 200 Protein: 18.5g Carbs: 18g Fiber: 3g Sugar: 3g Fat: 5.5g (Unsaturated: 4.5g Saturated: 1g)

Chicken and Olive Bake

SERVES 5 / PREP TIME: 10 MINUTES / COOK TIME: 5 HOURS HIGH/ 8 HOURS LOW

The tender chicken pairs really well with the saltiness of the olives.

1 tbsp olive oil
12oz skinless chicken breasts
2 slices of preserved lemon
½ cup pitted black olives, whole
2 tsp dried cilantro
2 tsp cumin
1 cup low FODMAP vegetable stock
1 tbsp low sodium tomato paste

1. Brown the chicken over medium-high heat in a little olive oil.
2. Add the chicken to the slow cooker.
3. Add in the rest of the ingredients and stir together well.
4. Cover and cook on High for 5 hours or Low for 8 hours.
5. Serve alongside your choice of rice or quinoa.

Hint: If you're watching your sodium intake you can rinse the olives before cooking.)

Hint: As this meal serves 8, portion up the leftovers and freeze in an airtight container for 2-3 weeks.

Per serving: Calories: 157 Protein: 21g Carbs: 2g Fiber: 1g Sugar: 1g Fat: 7g (Unsaturated: 6g Saturated: 1g)

Tunisian Chicken

SERVES 8 / PREP TIME: 10 MINUTES / COOK TIME: 5 HOURS HIGH/ 8 HOURS LOW

Nicely spiced and full of flavor.

4x 5oz chicken breast fillets
2 white potatoes, peeled and cut into
1in cubes
2 carrots, peeled and cut into 1in cubes
1 tbsp olive oil
1 stalk of celery, sliced
1 tsp cumin
1 tsp turmeric
1 tbsp fresh cilantro

1 lemon, quartered
1 cup beef tomatoes, quartered

1. Brown the chicken over medium-high heat in a little olive oil.
2. Keep the lemon and tomatoes to one side for now.
3. Into the slow cooker, add the chicken with the rest of the ingredients and stir well.
4. Cover and cook on High for 5 hours or Low for 8 hours.
5. Add the tomatoes for the last hour.
6. Serve alongside rice with a wedge of lemon.
7. Finish by garnishing with a scattering of fresh cilantro.

Hint: As this meal serves 8, portion up the leftovers and freeze in an airtight container for 2-3 weeks.

Per serving: Calories: 150 Protein: 17g Carbs: 11.5g Fiber: 2g Sugar: 1.5g Fat: 4g (Unsaturated: 3g Saturated: 1g)

Tangy Orange Chicken

A classic combination of citrus and juicy chicken.

2 tbsp olive oil
4 5oz boneless skinless chicken breasts
2 cup water
1 fresh orange, sliced
1 tsp dried cilantro
2 cups low FODMAP chicken stock
4 slices of preserved lemon
½ cup fresh parsley, chopped

1. Heat the oil in a skillet over medium heat.
2. Season the chicken and add to the pan.
3. Sauté for 4 minutes each side until browned all over.
4. Remove and set aside.
5. Into the slow cooker add the water, orange slices, cilantro and stock.
6. Stir in the chicken and preserved lemon.
7. Cook on Low for 7-8 hours or High for 4-5 hours.
8. Finish by garnishing with a little bit of parsley.

Hint: As this meal serves 8, portion up the leftovers and freeze in an airtight container for 2-3 weeks.

Per serving: Calories: 135 Protein: 17.5g Carbs: 3g Fiber: 0.5g Sugar: 1.5g Fat: 5.5g (Unsaturated: 4.5g Saturated: 1g)

SOUPS AND STOCKS

Slow Cooker Chicken Soup

SERVES 4 / PREP TIME: 10 MINUTES / COOK TIME: 6 HOURS LOW

This classic dish tastes wonderful after cooking all day—and smells good too!

Olive oil cooking spray
1 lb skinless chicken breasts
2 large carrots, peeled and chopped
2 parsnips, peeled and chopped
1/2 cup chives (green tips only), finely chopped
2 tbsp garlic-infused oil
1 tbsp fresh lemon juice
1/2 tsp dried thyme
1/2 tsp dried rosemary

1/2 tsp dried oregano
2 dried bay leaves
4 cups low FODMAP chicken stock
A pinch of salt to taste
3 tbsp fresh parsley, finely chopped
1 tbsp fresh cilantro, chopped

1. Spray the slow cooker dish with cooking spray.
2. Line the bottom of the slow cooker with the chicken breasts.
3. Cover with the carrots, parsnips, chives, garlic-infused oil, fresh lemon juice, thyme, rosemary, oregano, and bay leaves.
4. Cover everything with the low FODMAP chicken stock.
5. Season with a pinch of salt to taste.
6. Place the lid on the slow cooker.
7. Cook on Low for 6 hours.
8. Just before serving, remove chicken, allow to cool and shred using two forks.
9. Return to the soup and stir well.
10. Dish the hot chicken soup into bowls and sprinkle with the parsley and cilantro to serve.

Per serving: Calories: 276 Protein: 32g Carbs: 20g Fiber: 4g Sugar: 6g Fat: 8g

Warming Potato Soup

SERVES 8 / PREP TIME: 10 MINUTES / COOK TIME: 6-7 HOURS LOW

Perfect for cold days to warm you up.

---

5 medium baking potatoes, peeled and cubed (4-5 cups)
2 large carrots, thinly sliced in rounds
1 tbsp olive oil
1 tbsp butter
1/2 tsp salt
1/2 tsp ground black pepper

2 cups low FODMAP chicken stock
1/2 cup cottage cheese
2 tbsp cornstarch/potato starch

---

1. Place first 7 ingredients in the slow cooker, stirring well.
2. Cover and cook on Low for 6-7 hours.
3. When ready to serve, add the cheese.
4. Stir until lumps dissolve.
5. To thicken the soup, add the starch and stir well.

Hint: If you prefer a thinner soup, leave the starch out.

Per serving: Calories: 193 Protein: 5g Carbs: 26g Fiber: 3g Sugar: 2g Fat: 8g (Unsaturated: 2g Saturated: 5g)

Wholesome Tomato Pasta Soup

SERVES 5 / PREP TIME: 5 MINUTES / COOK TIME: 4 HOURS HIGH/8 HOURS LOW

An old-time favorite with a little something extra.

---

28 oz canned tomatoes
1 tsp olive oil
2 tbsp brown sugar
1 tsp dried oregano
1 tsp dried rosemary
1 tsp sea salt
1/2 tsp ground black pepper
6 cups low FODMAP chicken stock

1/2 cup tomato paste
3 cups cooked gluten free elbow macaroni

---

1. Add the tomatoes, oil, sugar, herbs, salt, pepper, and stock to your slow cooker pan.
2. Cook on High for 4 hours or Low for 8 hours.
3. 20 minutes before serving, mix in the tomato paste and the pasta.
4. Serve steaming hot in nice big bowls.

Per serving: Calories: 230 Protein:13g Carbs:40g Fiber: 9g Sugar: 15g Fat: 4g (Unsaturated: 3g Saturated: 1g)

Classic Creamy Tomato Soup

SERVES 5 /   PREP TIME: 5 MINUTES /   COOK TIME: 4 HOURS HIGH/8 HOURS LOW

Hot and delicious, perfect for a hot lunch or as a starter.

---

28 oz can of crushed tomatoes
4 cups low FODMAP chicken stock
1 tsp oregano
1 tbsp garlic-infused oil
1 tsp brown sugar
1 tsp ground black pepper
1 cup dairy free cream or rice milk

---

1. Add tomatoes, chicken stock, oregano and oil to the crock pot.
2. Add in the sugar and pepper.
3. Stir well.
4. Cook on High for 4 hours or Low for 8 hours.
5. Strain the soup and purée any chunks in a blender.
6. (Hint: You can also blend with an immersion blender for a very smooth consistency.)
7. Return the soup to the slow cooker.
8. Add cream/milk and stir well.

Per serving: Calories: 181 Protein: 6g Carbs: 12g Fiber: 3g Sugar: 8g Fat: 13g (Unsaturated: 4g Saturated: 9g)

Rustic Fish Stock

SERVES 8 / PREP TIME: 20 MINUTES / COOK TIME: 1 HOUR ON LOW

This works as a great base for noodle dishes, sauces or fish soups.

3 lb fish bones, including heads
10 cups water
3 green onion stalks, (green tips only)
chopped
2 zucchinis, roughly sliced

1. Place the fish bones and water to a large pan and bring to the boil over high heat.
2. Lower to medium and simmer for 20 minutes, then pass through a strainer into the slow cooker.
3. Add the vegetables to the slow cooker and cook on Low for 1 hour.
4. Strain again, then use straight away or store.

Hint: You can store stock in a sealable container in the fridge for up to 4 days. Otherwise, store it in portions in the freezer for 2-3 weeks.

Per serving: Calories: 65 Protein: 11g Carbs: 4g Fiber: 1g Sugar: 2g Fat: 1g (Unsaturated: 0g Saturated: 0g)

Low FODMAP Chicken Stock

SERVES 6 / PREP TIME: 10 MINUTES / COOK TIME: 6 HOURS ON LOW

Incredibly versatile, a great base for many recipes in this cookbook.

2-3 lb whole chicken (thighs, breasts and legs cut up)
2 celery stalks with leaves, diced
2 medium carrots, chopped
2 tsp dried thyme
2 green onion stalks, (green tips only) chopped

½ tsp dried oregano
10 whole black peppercorns
5-7 cups cold water (to fully cover ingredients)

---

1. Place all the ingredients in a large slow cooker.
2. Cover and cook on Low for 6 hours.
3. Gently remove the chicken from the stock and set aside.
4. Strain the stock and discard the vegetables.
5. (Hint: Alternatively, keep the vegetables and use them for a soup.)
6. Use immediately or store for later.
7. Once cooled, you can skim the fat from the surface to use.

Hint: You can store stock in a sealable container in the fridge for up to 4 days. Otherwise, store it in portions in the freezer for 2-3 weeks.

Per serving: Calories: 188 Protein: 24g Carbs: 4g Fiber: 1g Sugar: 1g Fat: 8g (Unsaturated: 5g Saturated: 2g)

Low FODMAP Vegetable Stock

SERVES 6 / PREP TIME: 5 MINUTES / COOK TIME: 6 HOURS ON LOW

A great veggie alternative for soups, sauces or as a base for many recipes.

2 celery stalks, roughly chopped
2 large carrots, roughly chopped
1 cup rutabaga, peeled and chopped
3 bay leaves
2 tsp dried oregano
2 sprigs of fresh rosemary
2 sprigs of fresh thyme
1 bunch fresh chives, chopped (green tips only)
5 whole black peppercorns

A pinch of salt
5-7 cups cold water (to fully cover ingredients)

1. Place all the ingredients into a large slow cooker.
2. Cover and cook on Low for 6 hours.
3. Skim the foam that may have risen to the top.
4. Pass the stock through a fine sieve.
5. Discard vegetables and herbs.
6. Allow to cool.

Hint: You can store stock in a sealable container in the fridge for up to 4 days. Otherwise, store it in portions in the freezer for 2-3 weeks.

Per serving: Calories: 26 Protein: 1g Carbs: 6g Fiber: 2g Sugar: 3g Fat:0g (Unsaturated: 0g Saturated: 0g)

VEGETARIAN

Indulgent Macaroni and Goats Cheese

SERVES 8 / PREP TIME: 10 MINUTES / COOK TIME: 3 HOURS LOW

A perfect bowl of comfort food; it's okay to treat yourself once in a while!

Olive oil cooking spray
1 egg white
½ lb dry gluten free macaroni (approx. 1/2 box)
2 ½ cups goat milk
2 tbsp unsalted butter, diced
2 cups goats cheese, crumbled

1. Spray the base and sides of your slow cooker with olive oil cooking spray.
2. (Hint: This keeps the macaroni from sticking to the sides of the cooker.)
3. Pour the beaten egg white into the slow cooker.
4. Add the dry macaroni.
5. Pour in the milk.
6. Add the butter.
7. Sprinkle in a little salt (if desired).
8. Crumble the cheese into the pot.
9. Stir the ingredients well to mix.
10. Cook on Low for 3 hours.

Per serving: Calories: 262 Protein: 14g Carbs: 25g Fiber: 1g Sugar: 2g Fat: 11g (Unsaturated: 7g Saturated: 8g)

Easy Jacket Potatoes

SERVES 6 / PREP TIME: 10 MINUTES / COOK TIME: 4 HOURS HIGH/8 HOURS LOW

A great lunch or side with your favorite topping.

---

6 large baking potatoes
1 ½ tbsp coconut oil
A pinch of celery salt to taste
Fresh ground pepper to taste
Your choice of low FODMAP topping

---

1. Scrub and dry the potatoes.
2. Pierce each potato a few times with a fork.
3. Rub each potato with a little coconut oil (use paper towel or your fingers).
4. Season with celery salt, and pepper and wrap in aluminum foil.
5. Place in the slow cooker.
6. Cook on High for 4 hours or Low for 8 hours.
7. Enjoy with a knob of butter or your choice of topping – goats cheese and tomatoes work well or you could try cottage cheese and chopped green chives with a squeeze of lemon.

(Without topping:)
Per serving: Calories: 246 Protein: 6g Carbs: 49g Fiber: 6g Sugar: 2g Fat: 4g
(Unsaturated: 0g Saturated: 3g)

Bubbling Tomato and Pepper Pasta Bake

SERVES 6 / PREP TIME: 10 MINUTES / COOK TIME: 3 HOURS LOW

A great plate of soft pasta in a rich Italian sauce.

4 cups gluten free pasta shapes of your choice
2 red bell peppers, diced
2 green bell peppers, diced
1 cup low FODMAP vegetable stock
2 cups beef tomatoes, diced
A pinch of salt and pepper
1 tsp dried oregano
1 tsp dried rosemary
3 cups fresh spinach

1. Add the pasta and peppers to the slow cooker and mix well.
2. Pour in the stock and beef tomatoes and stir to combine.
3. Sprinkle in the salt and pepper, then add the herbs.
4. Cook on High for 3 hours.
5. Add the spinach about 30 minutes before serving until wilted.
6. Spoon onto plates and enjoy.

Per serving: Calories: 312 Protein: 12g Carbs: 62g Fiber: 6g Sugar: 6g Fat: 2g (Unsaturated: 1g Saturated: 0g)

Root Vegetables, Quinoa and Herbs

SERVES 2 / PREP TIME: 5 MINUTES / COOK TIME: 5 HOURS LOW/1 HOUR HIGH

Winter vegetables with soft, tasty quinoa.

---

1 cup quinoa
1 cup beef tomatoes, coarsely chopped
1 tbsp dried oregano
1 tsp dried thyme
2 medium carrots, diced
½ rutabaga, peeled and diced
1 cup pumpkin, diced

A pinch of salt
1 cup water
1 cup fresh spinach

---

1. Add all the ingredients to the slow cooker and stir well.
2. Cook everything on Low for 5 hours or High for 1 hour, or until the quinoa has soaked up most of the liquid.
3. Serve and enjoy.

Hint: To speed up the cooking process you can soak the quinoa overnight in double the amount of water as quinoa. Reduce cooking time by half and leave out the water when cooking.

Per serving: Calories: 427 Protein: 16g Carbs: 82g Fiber: 16g Sugar: 16g Fat: 6g (Unsaturated: 4g Saturated: 1g)

Potato Dauphinoise

SERVES 5 / PREP TIME: 5 MINUTES / COOK TIME: 1-2 HOURS HIGH

Wonderfully creamy and perfect as a side or a casserole topping.

---

5 medium white potatoes, peeled and
thinly sliced
1 tbsp olive oil
2 tbsp potato starch
1 cup rice milk
1½ tsp salt
1 tsp dried parsley
A pinch of black pepper
1 tbsp fresh thyme

---

1. Start by layering the potatoes in the bottom of the slow cooker.
2. Make sure it's 3 layers deep and the base is fully covered.
3. For the béchamel, use a medium saucepan to heat the olive oil over medium-low heat until melted.
4. Add the potato starch and stir until smooth.
5. Cook until the mixture turns light golden, about 5 minutes.
6. Slowly add the milk to the mixture, whisking continuously until smooth.
7. Bring to a rolling boil over high heat.
8. Cook for 10 minutes over medium heat, stirring constantly, then remove from heat.
9. Season with salt, parsley and pepper.
10. Pour this over the potatoes in the slow cooker.
11. Cook on High for 1-2 hours until bubbling.
12. Finish with a scattering of fresh thyme.

Per serving: Calories: 153 Protein: 5g Carbs: 35g Fiber: 2g Sugar: 5g Fat: 1g
(Unsaturated: 1g Saturated: 0g)

Winter Stew with Parsnip and Fennel

SERVES 5 / PREP TIME: 5 MINUTES / COOK TIME: 4 HOURS LOW

Delicious and brilliantly simple.

---

2 cups low FODMAP vegetable stock
2 cups parsnip, peeled and cubed
3 or 4 collard green leaves, ribs
removed + chopped
5 small fennel hearts
1 tbsp garlic-infused oil
3 bay leaves
1 tsp turmeric

1 tsp dried parsley
A pinch of ground celery seed
A pinch of dried rosemary
A pinch of salt to taste
A pinch of coarse ground pepper, to taste

---

1. Combine all the ingredients and cook on Low for 4 hours (or until all the veggies are tender.)
2. Remove the bay leaves before spooning into bowls.

Per serving: Calories: 129 Protein: 5g Carbs: 23g Fiber: 7g Sugar: 9g Fat: 4g (Unsaturated: 3g Saturated: 1g)

Vegan Sweet and Sour

SERVES 5 / PREP TIME: 5 MINUTES / COOK TIME: 7 HOURS LOW

Delicious bold flavors, serve with rice or as a sauce for noodles.

2 ½ cups low FODMAP vegetable stock
2 cups water
1 tbsp tomato paste
2 tbsp extra virgin olive oil
4 stalks of celery, chopped
1 bok choy plant
1/2 cup carrots chopped
1 zucchini, diced
½ cup pineapple
A pinch salt and pepper

1. Heat the stock and water in a pan over high heat - bring to a boil.
2. Stir through the tomato paste.
3. Add the rest of the ingredients to the slow cooker.
4. Pour the liquid over the vegetables.
5. Cook on Low for 7 hours.

Per serving: Calories: 97 Protein: 3g Carbs: 10g Fiber: 3g Sugar: 6g Fat: 6g
(Unsaturated: 5g Saturated: 1g)

Quinoa and Slow Roasted Red Peppers

SERVES 8 / PREP TIME: 15 MINUTES / COOK TIME: LOW 8 HOURS/ HIGH 3 - 4 HOURS

Roasted peppers add a sweet, smoky taste to the quinoa.

---

2 medium red peppers
1 medium green pepper, diced (about 1½ cup)
4 cups low FODMAP vegetable stock
1 tsp dried oregano
2 tsp ground cumin
¼ tsp thyme
1 tsp sea salt

¾ cup uncooked quinoa, rinsed under cold water and drained
4 cup green beans, ends trimmed
8 lemon wedges
2 tbsp fresh cilantro, chopped

---

1. First, roast your peppers: turn the oven on to the highest broil setting.
2. Move the rack to about 1/3 of the way from the top of the oven.
3. Wash and dry the whole peppers and place them on a baking sheet.
4. Place in the oven and broil for 2-3 minute.
5. Make sure the tops are slightly blackened.
6. Turn them with tongs and continue broiling until most sides are blistered and blackened.
7. Remove the peppers from the oven.
8. Make a tent with a large piece of foil over the top of the peppers to let them sweat.
9. Meanwhile, add stock, oregano, cumin, thyme, and salt to the slow cooker.
10. Add quinoa and stir.
11. Carefully peel the skin off of the peppers.
12. Remove the stem and the seeds, too.
13. Dice and add to the slow cooker.
14. Stir gently to mix all of the ingredients together.
15. Cook on Low for 8 hours or on High for 3 - 4 hours or until the quinoa is tender.
16. Add in the green beans 30 minutes before the end.
17. Scoop into bowls and squeeze a lemon wedge over each serving before garnishing with cilantro to finish.

Per serving: Calories: 119 Protein: 5g Carbs: 20g Fiber: 4g Sugar: 4g Fat: 3g (Unsaturated: 1g Saturated: 2g)

Greek Olive and Pepper Rice

SERVES 8 / PREP TIME: 10 MINUTES / COOK TIME: 1 1/2 HOURS + 30 MINUTES HIGH

Soft, sweet peppers, salty olives and tasty rice.

2 tbsp garlic-infused olive oil
2 cups white rice
3 cups low FODMAP vegetable stock
4 cups water
1 red bell pepper, seeds removed and finely chopped
1 green bell pepper, seeds removed and finely chopped
1 tsp dried rosemary

1 ½ cups goats cheese
3/4 cup sliced black olives, pitted
2 tbsp fresh-squeezed lemon juice
A pinch of salt and fresh-ground black pepper to taste
1/4 cup sliced green onions (green tips only)

1. Heat the olive oil in a large heavy frying pan over medium heat.
2. Add the rice and sauté for 5 minutes, or until the rice is nicely browned.
3. Put the browned rice into the slow cooker.
4. Add the stock and water to the pan to remove any browned bits.
5. Add the de-glazed mixture to the cooker with the rice.
6. Cook on High for 1 ½ hours.
7. After 1 ½ hours add the peppers and cook for 15 minutes more.
8. Add in the rosemary at this point.
9. Add 1 cup of the cheese and all of the sliced olives to the slow cooker.
10. Cook for another 15 minutes.
11. Check the rice is cooked through, then stir in the lemon juice.
12. Season with salt and fresh-ground pepper to taste.
13. Top with additional crumbled goats cheese and green onions as desired.
14. Serve it hot.

Per serving: Calories: 306 Protein: 11g Carbs: 37g Fiber: 1g Sugar: 2g Fat: 13g
(Unsaturated: 6g Saturated: 6g)

SEAFOOD

Tomato and Olive Fish Stew

SERVING SIZE: 4 / PREP TIME: 10 MINUTES / COOK TIME: 7-8 HOURS LOW /3-4 HOURS HIGH

Delicate fish with the tang of capers and tomatoes.

4x 5oz white fish fillets
½ tsp capers
3 medium potatoes, sliced into 1cm/
half-inch thick slices
2 cups beef tomatoes, chopped
1 cup water

1 cup dry white wine
3 tbsp fresh parsley, chopped
½ cup pitted black olives
A pinch of sea salt
A pinch of oregano

1. Combine all ingredients in a slow cooker and cook on Low for 7-8 hours or High for 3-4 hours until fish is flaky.
2. Flake the fish fillets with a knife and fork and stir well.
3. Serve up with your choice of rice or potatoes.

Per serving: Calories: 304 Protein: 28g Carbs: 31g Fiber: 4g Sugar: 4g Fat: 3g (Unsaturated: 2g Saturated: 0g)

Spiced Fish Stew

SERVES: 6 / PREP TIME: 10 MINUTES / COOK TIME: LOW 7-8 HOURS/HIGH3-4 HOURS

Cod absorbs the delicious flavors it is cooked in.

2 tsp ground ginger
1 tsp ground cumin
1 tsp turmeric
1 lemon, juiced
2 cups fresh beef tomatoes, diced
1 tbsp chopped chives
1lb 2oz firm cod fillets
A pinch of salt and freshly ground

black pepper

1. Combine all ingredients in a slow cooker.
2. Cook on Low for 7-8 hours or High for 3-4 hours until fish is flaky.
3. Flake the cod fillets with a knife and fork and stir gently.
4. Serve with rice.

Hint: Season the fish with lemon, salt and pepper before cooking and leave to marinate over night if you have time.

Per serving: Calories: 79 Protein: 14g Carbs: 4g Fiber: 1g Sugar: 2g Fat: 1g (Unsaturated: 0g Saturated: 0g)

Spiced Shrimp Curry

SERVES 4 / PREP TIME: 10 MINUTES / COOK TIME: 1 HOUR + 15 MINUTES LOW

Succulent, spiced, meaty shrimp in a tomato and ginger based curry.

1 tsp cumin seeds
1 tsp coriander seeds
1 tsp fenugreek seeds
2 cups chopped tomatoes
1 thumb-sized piece of fresh ginger
1 tsp garlic-infused oil
1 tsp dried dill

1 cup low FODMAP vegetable stock
1 tbsp maple syrup
10½ oz shrimp, heads and shells removed, de-veined
1 tbsp lemon juice

1. For the curry sauce, heat a frying pan over medium heat.
2. Add the spices and dry fry for 2-3 minutes, or until fragrant.
3. Transfer the spices to a mortar and pestle and grind to a powder.
4. Add the tomatoes, ginger, garlic oil and dill to the slow cooker.
5. Add the stock and maple syrup and cook on Low for 1 hour.
6. Add the shrimp to the slow cooker and cook for a further 15-20 minutes on high or until shrimp is cooked through.
7. Serve with your choice of rice and a squeeze of fresh lemon.

Per serving: Calories: 139 Protein: 19g Carbs: 9g Fiber: 1g Sugar: 6g Fat: 3g
(Unsaturated: 3g Saturated: 0g)

Fresh Spanish-Inspired Mussels

SERVES 6 / PREP TIME: 10 MINUTES / COOK TIME: 2 HOURS + 10 MINUTES LOW

Deliciously tender mussels with a rich sauce.

---

1 red pepper, de-seeded and sliced
2 cups paella rice
1 cup chopped tomatoes
2 cups low FODMAP fish stock, heated through

1 cup fresh mussels (meat or in shell)
1 tbsp garlic-infused oil
1 tbsp dried parsley
1 tbsp freshly chopped parsley

---

1. Add the pepper and rice to the slow cooker and stir.
2. Stir in the chopped tomatoes with 2 cups of boiling water.
3. Add in the heated fish stock, cover, then cook on Low for 2 hours.
4. Uncover, then stir – the rice should have soaked up most of the liquid.
5. Stir in the mussels, garlic oil, and dried parsley.
6. (Hint: You can add a splash more water if the rice is looking dry.)
7. Cook for 10 minutes or until the mussels are cooked through.
8. Sprinkle with fresh parsley to serve in large bowls.

Hint: make sure to discard any mussels in the shell that don't open during or after cooking,

Per serving: Calories: 405 Protein: 20g Carbs: 58g Fiber: 3g Sugar: 5g Fat: 11g (Unsaturated: 8g Saturated: 2g)

Shrimp in Sweet and Sour Broth

SERVES 2 / PREP TIME: 10 MINUTES / COOK TIME: 40 MINUTES LOW + 10 MINUTES

These distinctive sweet and sour flavors complement the shrimp well.

3 tbsp rice vinegar or white wine vinegar
2 cups low FODMAP chicken stock
1 tbsp gluten free soy sauce
1 tbsp maple syrup

1 tsp ground ginger
3 green onions (green tips only), thinly sliced
½ cup canned pineapple, diced and juices drained
6 oz small raw peeled shrimp

1. Add the vinegar, stock, soy sauce, syrup and ginger to the slow cooker.
2. Add the green onions and cook on Low for 40 minutes
3. The sauce should have thickened by this point.
4. Add in the pineapple and heat through for 10 minutes.
5. Add the shrimp for 5 minutes or until thoroughly cooked through.

Per serving: Calories: 187 Protein: 21g Carbs: 20g Fiber: 1g Sugar: 12g Fat: 3g (Unsaturated: 2g Saturated: 1g)

Lemon and Cilantro Salmon

SERVES 6 / PREP TIME: 5 MINUTES / COOK TIME: 1 1/2 HOURS HIGH

Zesty and juicy salmon on a bed of soft rice.

---

1 lb salmon fillet, cut into 4 meal size portions
1 tsp salt and pepper
2 lemons, juice
2 tbsp fresh cilantro, finely chopped
½ cup cooked green beans to serve
1 cup cooked white rice

---

1. Line a piece of parchment paper into the slow cooker base.
2. Place the 4 salmon fillets flat on the parchment paper.
3. Sprinkle each with a little salt and pepper over the top.
4. Drizzle lemon juice over the salmon pieces and sprinkle with chopped cilantro.
5. Set on High and cook for 1 hour or 1 ½ hours for thicker cuts.
6. Once salmon is cooked, carefully lift out of the slow cooker.
7. Place into a shallow serving dish.
8. Remove the skin and serve.
9. Plate up with green beans and rice.

Per serving: Calories: 153 Protein: 20g Carbs: 10g Fiber: 1g Sugar: 1g Fat: 3g
(Unsaturated: 2g Saturated: 1g)

Slow-Cooked Calamari

SERVES 4 /　PREP TIME: 5 MINUTES /　COOK TIME: 20 MINUTES LOW

Calamari is rich in copper and selenium – two essential vitamins that work as antioxidants in your body. This serving alone contains more than your daily requirement of copper – great if you're lacking on other days!

---

8 oz raw calamari
1 medium yellow pepper, diced
1 ½ large red peppers, diced
1 cup green beans
1 tbsp coconut oil
1 tbsp freshly chopped parsley
1 cup water
1 tsp salt

---

1. Add all ingredients to a slow cooker , stir and cook on Low for 20-25 minutes or until calamari is cooked through but not over done.
2. Serve hot!

Hint: Take care not to over eat calamari, as it is also high in sodium – everything in moderation!

Per serving: Calories: 111 Protein: 10g Carbs: 8g Fiber: 2g Sugar:2g Fat: 5g (Unsaturated: 2g Saturated: 3g)

Seafood Bisque

SERVES 6 / PREP TIME: 5 MINUTES / COOK TIME: 4 HOURS LOW + 1 HOUR

A tasty mix of seafood with a herby sauce.

---

1 ½ cups chopped beef tomatoes
2 cups low FODMAP chicken/fish stock
2 celery stalks, finely sliced
1 medium red bell pepper, finely chopped
1 tsp dried thyme
8 oz crab meat, fresh or frozen
7 oz large size raw shrimp, rinsed

---

1. Tip in the tomatoes, stock and vegetables to the slow cooker.
2. Add the thyme and cook for 4 hours on Low.
3. (Hint: If you're in a rush, cook for 2 hours on High.)
4. Add the crab meat and shrimp and cook for another hour on Low.
5. Remove from the heat and serve.

Per serving: Calories: 123 Protein: 18g Carbs: 6g Fiber: 1g Sugar: 3g Fat: 2g
(Unsaturated: 2g Saturated: 0g)

Shrimp and Yellow Pepper Jambalaya

SERVES 6 / PREP TIME: 10 MINUTES / COOK TIME: 7 HOURS + 1 HOUR LOW

A vibrant and tasty dish.

---

1 lb uncooked peeled shrimp
4 cups cooked brown rice
28 oz diced beef tomatoes
1 cup chopped yellow bell pepper
1 tbsp parsley
1 cup chopped celery stalks
¼ tsp ground black pepper
½ tsp chopped chives
½ tsp sea salt

---

1. Hold the shrimp and rice to one side.
2. Place all the other ingredients into a slow cooker.
3. Cover and cook for 7 hours on Low. Add in the shrimp, rice and 8 cups water.
4. Cover and cook for another hour on Low.
5. Alternatively cook on High for 4 hours and then add the shrimp for 30 minutes on High.
6. Serve hot.

Per serving: Calories: 184 Protein: 14g Carbs: 27g Fiber: 4g Sugar: 7g Fat: 2g (Unsaturated: 2g Saturated: 0g)

Thai Clams with Rice

SERVES 8 / PREP TIME: 5 MINUTES / COOK TIME: 4 HOURS + 50 MINUTES LOW

A delicious Thai infused clam dish with ginger and lime.

---

2 medium yellow bell peppers, sliced
1 ½ cups rice
10 slices of grated fresh ginger peeled
32 oz low FODMAP fish stock
14 oz almond milk
¼ cup sliced green onions (green tips only)

2 cups fresh green beans, ends trimmed
15 oz fresh clams
1/3 cup fresh lime juice

---

1. Place the bell peppers, rice, and ginger into the slow cooker.
2. Pour in the fish stock and milk.
3. Stir well, cover and cook for 4 hours on Low or 2 hours on High.
4. Add the green onions and green beans.
5. Stir in the clams and lime juice.
6. Cover and cook for another 50 minutes on Low.
7. Transfer into serving bowls and enjoy.

Per serving: Calories: 164 Protein: 6g Carbs: 31g Fiber: 1g Sugar: 4g Fat: 2g
(Unsaturated: 1g Saturated: 0g)

DRINKS AND DESSERTS

Quick-Blitzed Banana Smoothie

SERVES 1 / PREP TIME: 5 MINUTES / COOK TIME: NA

Cold, refreshing and nutritious.

1/2 banana, peeled and sliced
½ cup almond milk
Handful of ice
1 tbsp maple syrup (optional)
1/2 tsp ground nutmeg

---

1. Place all of the ingredients into a blender.
2. Blitz until smooth.
3. Transfer to a serving glass and serve at once.

Per serving: Calories: 157 Protein: 1g Carbs: 35g Fiber: 2g Sugar: 29g Fat: 2g
(Unsaturated: 2g Saturated: 0g)

Raspberry and Cranberry Juice Blend

SERVES 2 / PREP TIME: 5 MINUTES / COOK TIME: NA

Deliciously refreshing.

---

1 cup cranberry juice
½ cup frozen organic raspberries, defrosted
Cup rice milk
1 tbsp brown sugar, or to taste
2 mint sprigs, to serve

---

1. Place all the ingredients into a blender and pulse until smooth.
2. Pour into glasses and serve topped with fresh mint.

Per serving: Calories: 156 Protein: 4g Carbs: 32g Fiber: 4g Sugar: 25g Fat: 2g (Unsaturated: 2g Saturated: 0g)

Blueberry Pancake Shake

SERVES 2 / PREP TIME: 5 MINUTES / COOK TIME: NA

Sweet and delicious - a real treat.

½ cup organic blueberries
1 tbsp maple syrup
1 tsp vanilla extract
1 cup almond milk

---

1. In a blender, add all the ingredients and blitz them up.
2. Pour into milkshake glasses and enjoy.

Per serving: Calories: 100 Protein: 1g Carbs: 20g Fiber: 1g Sugar: 18g Fat: 1g (Unsaturated: 1g Saturated: 0g)

Classic Strawberry Shake

SERVES 1 / PREP TIME: 5 MINUTES / COOK TIME: NA

Perfect to satisfy any milkshake cravings.

1/2 cup crushed ice
½ cup rice milk
1/2 banana, peeled and sliced
3 strawberries, halved
Handful of organic strawberries, plus
extra to garnish

---

1. Add ice to blender and pulse until you get fine pieces.
2. While ice is being crushed, measure the rice milk.
3. Add the milk and fruit and blend for approximately 1 minute or until smooth.
4. Serve.

Per serving: Calories: 132 Protein: 2g Carbs: 30gg Fiber: 4g Sugar: 20g Fat: 2g
(Unsaturated: 1g Saturated: 0g)

Rhubarb and Strawberry Crumble

SERVES 6 / PREP TIME: 10 MINUTES / COOK TIME: 2 1/2 HOURS HIGH

Fantastically tart and sweet with crumbly oaty topping.

3 cups organic strawberries, sliced
3 cups rhubarb, sliced
½ cup sugar
1 tbsp lemon zest
1 cup gluten free oats
¼ tsp ground nutmeg
½ cup very ripe banana, mashed

1. In a slow cooker, toss together the strawberries, rhubarb, sugar and lemon zest.
2. In a medium bowl, stir together the oats and nutmeg.
3. Mix in the mashed banana with your fingertips, crumbling until large 'breadcrumbs' are formed.
4. Heap this on top of the strawberry and rhubarb mixture.
5. Cover and cook on High for 2 ½ hours or until fruit is bubbling
6. Your topping will be crisp and lightly golden brown.
7. Spoon into bowls and enjoy.

Per serving: Calories: 178 Protein: 3g Carbs: 43g Fiber: 6g Sugar: 24g Fat: 1g
(Unsaturated: 0g Saturated: 0g)

Tropical Fruit Crumble

SERVES 6 / PREP TIME: `0 MINUTES / COOK TIME: 2 1/2 HOURS HIGH

Classic crumble with an exotic twist.

1 tsp olive oil
3 cups sliced mandarin, orange and
pineapple
3 nectarines, sliced
¼ cup sugar
2 tbsp rice flour
1 tsp grated lemon peel
2 tbsp brown sugar
¼ tsp ground nutmeg
¼ cup very ripe banana, mashed

1. Lightly oil the bottom of your slow cooker.
2. Add the mandarin, nectarines, sugar, rice flour and lemon peel, and toss them together.
3. In a medium bowl, mix the brown sugar, nutmeg, and banana.
4. Cut in the banana with a pastry blender or by criss-crossing two knives until the mixture looks like coarse sand.
5. You should be able to pinch the mixture and have it hold its shape.
6. Scatter the mixture over the top of the fruit.
7. Cover and cook on High for 2½ hours until the fruit is bubbling.
8. Spoon into bowls and serve hot.

Per serving: Calories: 127 Protein: 2g Carbs: 31g Fiber: 3g Sugar: 25g Fat: 0g
(Unsaturated: 0g Saturated: 0g)

Creamy Rice Pudding

SERVES 8 / PREP TIME: 10 MINUTES / COOK TIME: 3 HOURS LOW

A family favorite - warming and sweet.

---

3 cups cooked dessert rice
8 tbsp raisins
1 tsp vanilla extract
1 ½ cups coconut milk
1 tbsp sugar
1 tsp ground cinnamon

---

1. Line your slow cooker with a little coconut oil.
2. Mix all the ingredients except sugar and cinnamon in the slow cooker.
3. Cover and cook on Low for 3 hours.
4. The liquid should be absorbed by this point.
5. Stir the pudding.
6. Sprinkle with the sugar and the cinnamon to finish.
7. Serve warm.

Per serving: Calories: 216 Protein:3g Carbs: 28g Fiber: 2g Sugar: 9g Fat: 11g
(Unsaturated:1g Saturated: 10g)

CONVERSION TABLES

Volume

Imperial	Metric
1 tbsp	15ml
2 fl oz	55 ml
3 fl oz	75 ml
5 fl oz (¼ pint)	150 ml
10 fl oz (½ pint)	275 ml
1 pint	570 ml
1 ¼ pints	725 ml
1 ¾ pints	1 liter
2 pints	1.2 liters
2½ pints	1.5 liters
4 pints	2.25 liters

Oven temperatures

Gas Mark	Fahrenheit	Celsius
1/4	225	110
1/2	250	130
1	275	140
2	300	150
3	325	170
4	350	180
5	375	190
6	400	200
7	425	220
8	450	230
9	475	240

Weight

Imperial	Metric
½ oz	10 g
¾ oz	20 g
1 oz	25 g
1½ oz	40 g
2 oz	50 g
2½ oz	60 g
3 oz	75 g
4 oz	110 g
4½ oz	125 g
5 oz	150 g
6 oz	175 g
7 oz	200 g
8 oz	225 g
9 oz	250 g
10 oz	275 g
12 oz	350 g

BIBLIOGRAPHY

FODMAP food list (2017) Available at: http://www.ibsdiets.org/FODMAP-diet/FODMAP-food-list/ (Accessed: 22 February 2017).

Micawber (no date) Dangers of avoidance. Available at: http://www.ibs-health.com/page284.html (Accessed: 22 February 2017).

Ross, E. and Lam, M. (2016) 'The low FODMAPS diet and IBS: A winning strategy', Journal of Clinical Nutrition and Dietetics, 02(01). doi: 10.4172/2472-1921.100013.

Camilleri, M. and Acosta, A. (2014) 'Re: Halmos et al, A diet low in FODMAPs reduces symptoms of irritable bowel syndrome', Gastroenterology, 146(7), pp. 1829–1830. doi: 10.1053/j.gastro.2014.01.071.

Gibson, P.R., Varney, J.E. and Muir, J.G. (2016) 'Diet therapy for irritable bowel syndrome: Is a diet low in FODMAPS really similar in efficacy to traditional dietary advice?', Gastroenterology, 150(4), pp. 1046–1047. doi: 10.1053/j.gastro.2015.10.053.

Piacentino, D., Rossi, S., Piretta, L., Badiali, D., Pallotta, N. and Corazziari, E. (2016) 'Tu1425 role of FODMAPs, and benefit of Low-FODMAP diet, in irritable bowel syndrome severity', Gastroenterology, 150(4), p. S901. doi: 10.1016/s0016-5085(16)33048-7.

Chung, C.-Y. and Joo, Y.-E. (2014) 'Can a diet low in Fermentable Oligosaccharides, Disaccharides, Monosaccharides and polyols (FODMAPs) reduce the symptoms of irritable bowel syndrome?', The Korean Journal of Gastroenterology, 64(2), p. 123. doi: 10.4166/kjg.2014.64.2.123.

BS: Risk of IBS increases after bacterial infection (2015) Nature Reviews Gastroenterology and Hepatology, 12(6), pp. 313–313. doi: 10.1038/nrgastro.2015.86.

Sidebar (1998) Available at: http://www.aboutibs.org (Accessed: 23 February 2017).

INDEX

Made in the USA
Columbia, SC
13 December 2017